Powerful Life-Changing Hacks That Truly Transformed My Life

Simple yet effective hacks to transform physical, mental and emotional health rapidly and sustainably

Dr Mehmet Yildiz

Second Edition, September 2019

Copyright © Dr Mehmet Yildiz

Publisher: S.T.E.P.S. Publishing Australia

P.O Box 2097, Roxburgh Park, Victoria, 3064 Australia

info@stepsconsulting.com.au

Edited by FirstEditor.com

Disclaimer

Table of Contents

Contents

Chapter 1 – Introduction

Purpose of this book

The purpose of this book is to share what I learnt and practised recently to transform myself from multiple angles in my life. The emphasis is on the small changes which make a big impact on this journey.

The small changes presented in this book became a tipping point for me. Even though they look small and uninteresting from the outside, turning them into habits and combining them with each other made a remarkable transformation for my life.

I want to share the reasons behind trying these changes with no shame and explain how these changes helped me genuinely, using several examples from my personal life.

As the book is about my functional changes, I used the first-person narration of a conversational language rather than a formal style. I deliberately did not provide any citations to keep the book simple to read and comprehend. I know from my experience that cluttered citations in these types of practical books bore and turn off the readers.

If you want to delve into details, you can use the search terms related to the topics provided in the book. In this case, highlighted terms, tools, supplements, approaches, methods, and concepts provided in this book can easily be Googled, and relevant articles can easily be accessed from PubMed and other prominent scientific information sources.

The focus of this book

Unusually, the focus of this book is me as a person who tested several approaches based on trial and error and input from developing research. However, while writing, I thought about you as my audience to simplify my thoughts and add an order to my madness to make sense and add value to your life. So the focus of this book is You and I.

In this book, I don't make any recommendations on purpose. The reasons for this is that I aim to share my experience sincerely, without any hype or any motives other than utilitarian perspective and charitable goals.

However, I aim to share this experience with you, assuming that you may have a critical review of those points. I am hoping some readers can customise or apply some of the techniques based on their experience and needs. I deliberately make no recommendations for using these techniques.

Some readers may use them as a validation point as I did. I believe some readers are already using some of these techniques and approaches; hence, they keep nodding their heads and keep asking what is next.

Due to the controversial nature of some points, I believe some readers may be judging them and only after some hardships do they attempt to try relevant ones as a last resort.

We are all individuals and have different needs, expectations and circumstances. Therefore, I do not take any offence at any reaction. My genuine intention is to provide a practical perspective to my readers based on my experience, especially hard-learned lessons so that they can benefit as they become relevant and possible for their conditions.

Audience

The intended audiences for this book are those open-minded people who take personal responsibility and take action to transform themselves to their best version, leveraging the experience of others, tested bio-hacks, and proven tactics documented in an edited book format.

Forewarning

This book is not an advice or prescription to anyone. I only share my personal experience and findings. The points discussed in this book are publicly available in easily accessible knowledge sources such as PubMed.

Upfront, I am not a medical doctor, dietician, nutritionist or psychologist. However, I have professional doctoral and other post-doctoral degrees; hence, I can undertake advanced research and interpret the advanced studies. I am sort of a PubMed enthusiast as my hobby.

It is essential to state that this book can be read as a transformational biography of a person who tried different techniques and approaches which worked for his transformational goals.

I don't particularly recommend any of my transformational tools, techniques, approaches or personal hacks to anyone in this book, as every one of us is unique. The techniques I used may or may not work for other people. It is up to the discretion of the readers.

If you are open-minded like me and enjoy learning from other people's transformational stories, you may love this book and find it insightful. It truly reflects genuine thoughts, feelings and experiences in a long and painful journey.

However, it is vital to communicate upfront that if you take offence from people bio-hacking themselves, trying alternative approaches to the mainstream, eating dead animals from nose to tail, and renewing themselves relentlessly, this book may not be for you. There are many conservative and mainstream-oriented books for transformational goals.

Approach and context

In this book, I provide a practical approach based on the substantial experience of my transformation to better versions of myself. Reading and learning from a vast array of research publications, especially PubMed, is one of my favourite intellectual activities. However, on purpose, I did not quote a review of resources, as citations may have turned the book into a scientific publication with cumbersome details.

This book is intentionally written in a conversational format to make it easy to read and understand. Almost no jargon was used; if any jargon was used for any reason, it is briefly explained and clarified.

To reiterate, this is not a science book; however, most of the hacks have some backing of science. Nothing was tested randomly but tested based on some hypothesis and the experience of others who also tried similar approaches. Some approaches presented in this book are well-known, but the value comes from the customised trial of those alternatives and presenting the personal results openly, with no bias or financial stake at hand.

This book was not funded or endorsed by any person or institution. The book represents a factual and biographical presentation of my transformational experiences.

Chapter 2: Joyful Exercise

I want to start with exercise as this made the most significant impact on my transformational change. Before you stop reading, the exercises introduced here, not the type which can strain you but to give you pleasure. I won't tell you to go to the gym every day and perspire hours carrying of heavyweight or swim at five o'clock in the morning. I only introduce enjoyable and convenient exercise; therefore, I named this chapter as "Joyful Exercise".

Trampoline

I came across trampolines when a new Trampoline Fitness centre opened in our suburb years ago. My young son was so much into it that he dragged us to the centre almost every day. He is now an adult with good muscle build.

One day I was so curious when he was jumping with his friends and participated in his session. It was amazing fun. I was reliving my childhood. Time passed so quickly that a one-hour session was like one minute. My heart rate, which I checked from my smartwatch, was showing that it was very elevated. I was in a euphoric state.

After an hour's jumping session, I felt great that night. My sleep was flawless. After that each time we took our son to the centre, I kept jumping with the kids. With this simple activity, my fitness increased substantially in a month or so.

After a while, we couldn't go to the centre due to his other extracurricular activities and educational commitments. I was missing the fun but was reluctant to go to a children's centre as an adult.

Then one day I saw an advertisement on YouTube about a trampoline company in the USA. They were shipping overseas. The ad inspired me, so I ordered a small trampoline for my study room.

It was more expensive than my other fitness gear, but it was one of the best investments and most useful hacks I have ever tried. This simple tool made a significant impact on my health. It became my best friend in the winter, especially on rainy days when I couldn't go out.

I learnt innovative ways to use indoor trampoline. There are times I watch some programs on my PC or listen to Audible books. Those are the times to hop on the trampoline and slowly walk or jump on it. It helps me reduce my stress and complete my daily ten thousand step walking goal.

In addition, I learnt it has some additional benefits to our health. After learning those benefits, I observed the positive changes in my health. For example, it increases lymphatic flow in our bodies, hence helping detoxification. Cleansing the lymphatic system also can improve our immune system.

Another benefit I found in the literature was increased skeletal and overall bone density. This is extra important for my aging body. It can be preventative for skeletal decay.

Besides improved fitness, I also observed that my heart rate does not go as high as in my earlier days. Obviously, it helped me become fitter.

I also read about the benefit of increasing oxygen circulation, hence increasing cell energy. I don't have a device to test this, but my overall breathing profile improved based on the way I breathe during the trampoline sessions and even get better afterwards.

I used to run and jog years ago and used to feel awful afterwards due to pain in my joints. Now jogging, running or hopping on the trampoline, there is no excessive pressure on my joints. Protecting our joints is another preventative measure for premature aging and potential skeletal risks of disease.

Another benefit I gained from jumping on the trampoline in different patterns that I learnt from kids was gaining better balance. I read in the literature that jumping on a trampoline can stimulate the vestibular and the semicircular canals in the middle ear and help us improve balance.

Interestingly, some trampoline fans even make claims that it can prevent cancer through the improved circulation of the lymphatic fluid by removing cancerous cells in the body, but I don't have a way to test this in my hacks. However, it is refreshing to hear about these useful speculations as they may be validated in the future and become a truth. I'd personally keep an open mind about these potential benefits of trampolines.

Best of all, I did not experience any side effects of hopping on a trampoline. The only risk is falling from the trampoline if not done correctly or not paying attention. Therefore, I ensure that there are no sharp objects around the trampoline, and it is on a smooth carpet in my study room.

Vibration Machine

This wonder machine is excellent for overall muscle workout. It is fun and affordable. I usually hop on it for ten minutes and feel that all muscles are worked out. It was originally designed for the astronauts to keep muscle mass in space, as the fast vibration causes involuntary movements in muscles.

Since I started using a vibration machine, over twelve years now, I noticed improvements in my muscle tone and bone density.

Using a vibration machine daily also improved my fitness for other cardiovascular exercises. It has also been useful to maintain better balance, improved flexibility and coordination. Using a vibration machine with a trampoline at home has been the best combination of a daily exercise regimen for me even if I cannot go out or to the gym some days due to weather conditions, work schedule or other commitments.

Pull-up Machine

I found the pull-up machine a most effective strength and weight training tool. Pull-ups can be used to develop strength and increase muscle mass, focusing on the large muscles of the back and the biceps.

Having a pull-up machine at home and doing a few pull-ups in the mornings and the evenings after work turned into a good habit for me. On the days I cannot go to the gym, this pull-up machine, after the trampoline and vibration machine, is my first go-to machine at home. While using the trampoline and vibration machine for cardiovascular purposes, I use the pull-up machine for strength training.

Initially I was able to do only five pull-ups with great

difficulty. All my body was shaking and getting sore after even one set of five reps. After years of practice at home on my pull-up machine, I can now achieve 20 consecutive pull-ups daily with no recovery time required. It takes only five minutes to do three sets. I feel great when I perform three sets of 20 pull-ups in the morning. Purchasing a pull-up machine was only a $200 investment, but it was worth it.

Chapter 3: Fun Outdoor Practice

Smart Sun Exposure

For many years I feared the sun, especially living in the Southern hemisphere. Many scary ads on TV, showing people getting melanoma quickly from sun exposure were very discouraging for me. The ads were emphasising the lack of smartness in staying under the sun naked. They were not even pointing out the use of the sun for a short period. It was a binary guide, as the sunlight was evil. I had difficulty in believing these ads but complied with it for many regretful years.

I learnt that the ultraviolet-B radiation in sunlight was needed for the formation of Vitamin D in our bodies. Medical literature shows Vitamin D as a significant hormone-like ingredient for our health. It is proven that Vitamin D is preventative for inflammation, improves brain function, lowers high blood pressure, relaxes muscles, and even protects against some cancers, contrary to the message in the scary ads.

In addition to this piece of knowledge, I also thought that for thousands of years our ancestors were walking under the sun so our genes must be adapted to sunlight. This assumption made me act brave. I was determined to take personal responsibility on this risk.

With this motivational thought, and seeing many people using the sun in smart ways, I took the plunge to stay under the sunlight 15 minutes a day and increased it to 30 minutes after a while, exposing over 40 per cent of my body to the sun. For one year, using a 30-minute sunlight therapy made a tremendous positive difference for my health.

First, my Vitamin D levels reached an optimal level, as described by my family doctor. My testosterone level increased substantially. My cortisol level dropped to normal, as for many years it was elevated due to stress and inappropriate diets. My overwhelming inflammation, caused by arthritis, decreased substantially as evident from my blood inflation markers such as CRP. My mild depression and occasional insomnia disappeared, as I had a better hormonal balance. In short, my happiness and joy extended by exposing myself to sunlight 30 minutes a day.

I have been undertaking this regimen for over five years now. Regularly getting checked for potential risks such as melanoma, touch wood, I have experienced no side effects so far. My Vitamin D levels are still optimal, and I feel great when I see the sun, especially in the mornings. It is my first act to look at the sun a few minutes in the early morning to reset my circadian rhythm. This early morning sun exposure inhibits the melatonin production process; hence, drowsiness quickly disappears.

Since I started to perform this activity daily, I felt awake in the mornings and sleepy at nights. It is gratifying to follow a natural rhythm.

Barefoot Walk

Long ago, when our son started walking, our family nurse wanted him to start walking barefoot as it would help him perceive and be aware of the position and movement of his body with constant feedback. Later I found that this is called "proprioception" in the literature.

This piece of knowledge got stuck with me for years. I loved walking barefoot around the beach in the sand and on green grasses in parks and our garden. We maintain a clean and well-trimmed green grass in our backyard. Apart from looking appealing to the eye, it is my daily therapeutic tool.

Each time I walked on sand or grass barefoot, I felt some pleasantness in my body, as if the stress was melting away and replacing with enjoyable feelings.

One day I was curious and started reading about this and noticed that there is a massive trend for barefoot walking in various health communities. There were hundreds of anecdotes from people feeling good about barefoot walking, especially on sand and grass.

There were many testimonials on the benefits of walking barefoot on sand and grass, especially for reducing stress. Interestingly, I came across studies on this claiming stress reduction quantitatively, such as over 60%.

The most convincing argument for the benefit of walking on the sand or grass was related to electrons which can be transferred from our bodies. It was found out that negatively charged electrons from our body can be absorbed or neutralised by the earth.

This argument was convincing to me as I experienced the feeling by walking barefoot on grass and sand but also a piece of earthing equipment which I bought from eBay. Then I replicated this hack multiple times on other earthing products such as mats and bedsheets.

There is one caveat, though; those products, even though they made some changes in terms of good feelings, were not as effective as actual walks on sand or grass. Therefore, I made them supplementary sources of my earthing regimen on cold and rainy days when it becomes impossible to walk outside.

This earthing effect of barefoot had a tremendous effect on my sleep. On those days, I walked around the beach and, on the grass, I fell asleep quickly at night and stayed asleep longer. As mentioned in the sleep recording hack, checking my daily sleep patterns was empirical proof of the benefits of barefoot walking for good quality sleep.

My usual walking on sand or grass is around ten thousand steps a day. It has been very beneficial for my health from multiple angles such as keeping my weight, reserving my lean muscles and staying in a good mood. Slow walking around 90 minutes (ten thousand steps) is a habit that I developed over a decade and truly enjoyed every day. My smartwatch keeps me motivated to get the benefit of this good habit.

Another monitoring device in my smartphone is an app to measure my heart rate variability. When I read the claims that earthing improves heart rate variability, I tested it over six months and noticed a substantial improvement in my heart rate variability.

Besides these validated benefits, I read some testimonials and speculations such as improvement in cardiovascular health, autonomic nervous system balance, improvements in blood viscosity, and even boosting brainpower. They sound like amazing benefits, but I did not have a chance to validate them in my life yet. I am looking forward to seeing some convincing studies on these promising benefits.

Chapter 4: Instant Mental Boost

Cold shower

I never thought I was going to enjoy cold showers so much and replace my morning coffee with them. When I read the incredible benefits on a website many years ago, initially I thought it was just hype or exaggerated.

It created some curiosity in me, though, as I kept seeing various articles and YouTube videos about the benefits of cold showers. After reading several testimonials, one day, I decided to take a cold shower myself. It was the worst experience I ever had. My body reacted badly. I thought I was dying.

Then I watched YouTube videos on how others did it. I learned a bit about the techniques such as starting slowly with legs, arms, then head and whole body. The techniques I learnt helped me take cold showers a little easier.

However, what I learnt about how to deal with the body's response and the adaptation process was an eye-opener. Someone said that I wouldn't die in a few minutes of cold showers, even though the body feels like it. It is a survival mechanism of the body to react that way. In a few minutes, the body would get used to it and would start feeling good.

It was spot-on. After 30 seconds, my body got used to it. The adverse reaction slowly turned into positive. I started feeling better. The water seemed warmer after a while, even though I did not change the tap.

The best part was after the shower. It was a fantastic feeling. All lethargy and morning drowsiness disappeared in a few minutes. I felt as if I'd had three cups of strong espresso. Not only was my energy level high, but also, my confidence increased incredibly.

Nowadays, whenever I have a challenging day ahead, I have a few minutes of a cold shower and feel ready for the challenges of the day. This habit helped me reduce my coffee intake and caffeine dependence in the mornings.

After reading about the benefits of cold showers, one day, I discovered that having cold and hot showers together half an hour before bed can reset the circadian rhythm. This was beneficial information for me, as I frequently travelled over the Atlantic and like many other travellers, I used Melatonin to overcome my jetlag issues.

Trying 30 second cold and 30-second hot showers alternately five to ten times half an hour before bed did wonder in resolving my jetlag issues. I've since stopped using melatonin, as it has side effects such as feeling drowsy the next day, especially if it is a cloudy winter day.

Brain Games

As I studied cognitive science at the post-graduate level, I knew the importance of stimulating our brains using various methods. In addition to habitual reading, I also used various crossword puzzles, Sudoku and other mind exercises in books, especially from Mensa or other intelligence-oriented publications. These were all very helpful.

My discovery of Lumosity and Elevate made a real difference in stimulating my brain. Initially, I was a bit doubtful of the benefits touted by the owners of these products. After a while playing with them daily, I not only enjoyed the time spent on those creative brain games, but I also noticed an improvement in my memory, attention, flexibility and agility.

Both Lumosity and Elevate provide a progressive approach to brain games. Timing is an essential factor. They also challenge for speed.

I am looking forward to new games to challenge my working memory, retention, focus, and problem-solving. A daily ten minutes brain gym is a fantastic opportunity to keep our brains healthy and fit.

Mindfulness and Meditation

Mindfulness became a lifestyle for me. Practising mindfulness, on a daily basis, made the most significant impact on my mental and emotional health. Since I started practising mindfulness, my overall optimistic mood improved considerably. I behad a new personality.

Mindfulness is essential to me because I see instant benefits at the times when I genuinely get stuck and feel miserable. As soon as I start practising mindfulness by being in the moment, by being aware of the things around me, my emotions and sensations in my body, suddenly I can see a dramatic drop in my stress and anxiety.

I learnt to practice mindfulness anywhere, anytime. It is an effortless natural state. Many traditions use it in different formats under different names—for example, contemplative practices in prayer or mediation formats.

For me, the purest form of mindfulness is focusing on my breath as soon as I notice my brain is ruminating. I take a deep breath, counting to four, then hold it for a count of four, then release it to a count of four again. While doing this slow breathing rhythm for a few minutes, I keep focusing on each breath. Then I continue my natural breathing process and focus on each in, out and the space in between. Whenever a thought comes to my mind, I gently remind myself that my focus is on my breathing.

Practising this simple process for 20 minutes a day works best for me. I usually try ten minutes in the morning when I wake up and ten minutes before I go to bed at night.

Epsom Salts

Discovering the use of Epsom salts in my baths made a massive difference in my physical sensations. More specifically, Epsom salt, which is Magnesium Sulphate, helped relax my muscles, especially after a workout or a stressful situation.

In addition, having a bath with Epsom salts helped me sleep better, reduce my stress and increase my magnesium intake in a comfortable way. Sadly, magnesium in tablet or powder format, usually more than 600 mg, caused me to have diarrhoea. I take my magnesium tablets once a day an hour before sleep.

Having an Epsom salts bath is terrific, but I also use it as a solution spray for topical use at other times. It is easier to carry the spray where I go. Whenever I feel soreness in my muscles, I spray some Epsom salt water on them and feel the relaxation in a short time. It is an essential tool in my emergency bag.

Journaling

Journaling has been one of my best-established habits for many years. It became an extension of my brain and retention capability. I jot down anything important in my day in my electronic journal. Writing things give me significant relief.

It is straightforward to keep an electronic journal nowadays. Many smartphones, tablets and laptops have free text editors. You can simply jot down your thoughts, ideas, plans, and so on as they come to you.

As it is your journal, you don't have to worry about grammar, structure, or editing. It can be an informal way of writing your thoughts. Journaling is a viable option for everyone. If you don't have an electronic device, it is fine; you can journal in a notebook. In fact, handwriting on a piece of paper maybe even more therapeutic, as is pointed out in classic psychology literature.

Journaling allows me to clarify my thoughts and feelings, especially for problematic situations. Through journaling, I gain valuable self-knowledge and confidence.

In addition, I use it as a problem-solving tool. Interestingly, when I start using my keyboard on my laptop, my thoughts get more explicit, and solutions to my problems come to tips of my touch-typing fingers. It is almost like a spiritual act. I feel like my higher self is talking to me via my fingertips.

Blogging can be a kind of journaling. However, since blogging is shared publicly, we cannot write private matters in a blog. It can be useful to share general ideas and thoughts which are appropriate to share. However, in private journaling, we can write about everything in detail, without the risk of offending anyone except ourselves.

Self-Conversation

There are times that I enjoy talking to myself about a specific point that requires some personal insights. It can be a therapeutic or creative activity. This technique helped me to be an inventor and produce innovative solutions at work.

Sometimes I record my conversations using a smartphone or laptop. Google docs is a free tool I use for this purpose on my PC. In addition, as an added value, this free word processing software converts my recorded voice to text.

Then I can insert the converted text into my daily journal.

Listening to my recorded conversations later gives me clues about my mood and overall psychological situation during the recording time. This insightful information helps me recognize important patterns about my feelings and thoughts.

Through recording my self-conversations and analysing them daily, I am like my own therapist who can monitor himself and make necessary therapeutic adjustment as required. This helps me save therapy funds. In my opinion, being in control of one's mental and emotional health is a fascinating privilege in this life.

Besides, as English was my second language, I had the tremendous benefit of improving my conversational English by using this voice recording method. It has been fascinating to listen to my own voice, detect my own mistakes based on my grammar knowledge, and correct them for better usage and improved fluency. This lingual activity also contributes to my cognitive reserves, which is a broad topic beyond the scope of this book. I plan to share this experience in another book, perhaps in a more scientific one.

Uplifting Music

Like many people, I find music as a tool to instantly boost my mood. For many years, when I was studying, background instrumental music was my concentration tool. It was mainly baroque music that primarily facilitated my learning. I still listen to baroque music for relaxation and motivation.

In addition, when I am in a low mood for any reason, I listen to uplifting music from my selected best pieces in an extensive collection. It doesn't take too long to lift my mood to a positive state when I listen to those selected pieces. As potent reminders, they immediately send convincing signals to my brain to move from a negative to a positive zone.

Use of uplifting music in challenging times helped me to transform myself from a pessimistic to an optimistic person. I learnt that my brain was pessimistic as the default unless I made a special effort to move it to an optimistic state.

Another tool that I discovered was dancing, combined with my uplifting music, at times when I really feel lethargic. Just five to ten minutes of dancing with selected uplifting music provide an additional cognitive boost to my mind and a noticeable uplift to my body. My brain loves to dance and music and responds with favourable reactions. For example, has anyone seen Kerry Muzzey's "Architect of the Mind" with choreography by Christopher Scott on YouTube?

Chapter 5: Smart Sleep

Sleep Monitoring

Sleep is essential in our lives, both short term and long term. It plays an essential role in every aspect of our health. Everyone knows this and makes a conscious effort to sleep every night. Studies associate quality sleep with many benefits such as better mood, better memory, better libido, and lower cardiovascular risks.

I learnt the importance of sleep when I was very young and adopted the conventional wisdom of going to bed early and rising early. My aim has always been to get at least eight hours of sleep.

Until recently, I thought sleeping eight hours was enough, so I never suspected that my terrible weaknesses some days were related to sleep deprivation. Feeling sleepy after eight hours of sleep was a mystery to me.

The awakening moment happened when I purchased my first fitness smart-watch over five years ago. It was a Fitbit device. It was monitoring how many hours I slept, how many times I was restless and the quality percentage of my sleep. It was accessible from my phone, tablet or PC.

After a few days of monitoring my sleep, I noticed that even though I allocated eight hours for my sleep, I was sometimes having less than six hours of quality sleep. Two hours were recorded as awake or restless. It was devastating when I noticed that.

Then based on this information, I increased my sleep hours and ensured that the quality hours were at least eight hours. Then there was a massive change in my mood, energy level, and overall feel. I was feeling wonderful on those days when the quality sleep was recorded at eight hours or more. It was an important lesson to learn that not the total sleep hours, but the quality sleep hours mattered.

Another benefit of sleep monitoring is to see how long it takes to fall asleep. This small piece of information may have significant effects on establishing sleep patterns. If I cannot fall asleep in 20 minutes, I get up and try to perform some sleep-inducing activities as recommended by the CBT (Cognitive Behavioural Therapy) practices.

Nowadays, I consistently use my smart-watch to monitor my sleep daily. Every morning I check my Fitbit dashboard for the amount and quality of sleep I get. If for any reason I get less than eight hours of sleep I take informed actions to rectify.

Here is one key hack I learnt related to dealing with short-term sleep deprivation to be effective at work or whatever we were supposed to do that day. I use a supplement called N-Acetyl-Tyrosine with a caffeine tablet. Tyrosine is an amino acid, and this acetyl version can pass the brain-blood barrier. It helps me to stay alert at least six hours with good feelings. I rarely need to use it, but when I need it, it works wonders for me. I provided more about this in the supplement's sections.

Silicone Ear Plugs

I am susceptible to sound. Especially if any noise is made when I am in bed in the middle of the night, I wake up immediately. Even the smallest noises can wake me up quickly.

For many years, I didn't know why I was waking up so frequently. Once I learnt to use silicone earplugs to reduce noise coming to my ears, my sleep quality really improved.

After using the silicone earplugs, the frequency of my

wake-ups dramatically decreased. I tried a few different types of earplugs, but they were not as practical and comfortable as the silicone earplugs. They are cheap and easy to find in many pharmacies or online convenience stores.

Eye Mask

Darkness is essential for quality sleep. Our brains are wired to produce melatonin naturally when it gets dark. Therefore, sleeping in a dark room is very important to have a restful sleep.

Even though I keep my room dark, there are times some little light can enter the room through various means. As a secondary support scheme to maintain absolute darkness, I use black silk eye masks.

After using the silicon earplugs, and adding an eye mask to my sleep regimen, the quality of my sleep further improved. When I get quality sleep, my day proceeds smoothly, with optimism, joy and happiness. Even the most prominent challenges look manageable.

Cool Room

A cool room is another essential factor to maintain quality sleep. Long ago I thought that a warm, cosy room would be great to sleep but I was so wrong. It was counterintuitive.

Once I learned to reduce the temperature of my room around 18 Celsius degrees, my sleep quality improved further. Interestingly, my body got used to the cooler temperature.

The biggest problem with the warm room was waking up in the middle of the night with perspiration and a tender body. I hated to feel itchy at night, which used to cause me to lose sleep and make me an insomniac. Therefore, I warmly embraced the cool temperature in my bedroom.

Air Cleaner

In addition to the above practical measures, I also added an air cleaner to my bedroom after reading many positive testimonials on them.

Adding an air cleaning machine to my bedroom made me feel the difference in breathing fresh and clean air at night. Such an affordable, quiet machine is an ideal addition to the bedroom for improving quality of sleep.

In addition, I also added Himalayan salt-based lamps to my bedroom. These lamps are believed to spread negative ions, attracting positive toxic molecules in the air. However, I don't have a measure to prove the effectiveness of these lamps. They can be excellent additions to the bedroom. I like breathing clean air at home.

Cold and Hot Shower

Since I started having 30 seconds cold and 30 seconds hot shower for around three minutes before going to bed, I felt a big difference in falling asleep quickly and having a deep sleep.

My understanding of the mechanism for alternating cold and a hot shower before sleep is resetting the circadian rhythm.

I provide more information about my cold shower regimen and its benefits in the Cold Shower section in this book.

Blue Light Blocking

It is nice to have natural blue light exposure during the day. However, exposure to blue light at night can be problematic, as this exposure can adversely affect our circadian rhythm.

However, there are practical solutions to address these. One of the most effective solutions is using blue light blocking glasses. We can also turn off blue light-producing devices such as mobile phones, tablets, PCs and TVs at least an hour before we go to bed. Dimming lights and reducing blue light exposure even earlier, such as two to three hours before bed, is recommended.

As a practical implementation, I learnt to use flux software on my PC to address this issue at nights. My mobile phone also automatically goes to night shift light scheme.

After learning the adverse effect of blue light on the circadian rhythm, I removed all the blue light producing devices from my room. It was in many gadgets such as the alarm clock and even in my beloved air cleaning machine, so I cover its blue light with a piece of dark, sticky paper.

Optimised Magnesium

Taking a magnesium tablet an hour before my bedtime contributed to my sleep quality. The usual dose of magnesium I take is around 400 Mg. More than this caused diarrhoea for me. Because of the poor digestion of magnesium intake, I learnt to take magnesium through my skin.

Therefore, I take a bath with Epsom salts. This is the sulphate form of magnesium and well tolerated by the skin. In addition, sometimes, I use magnesium cream if there are any sore muscles in my body, especially on the days with strength training.

In addition to stress and relaxation of muscles, I learnt that optimized magnesium in our bodies has many other benefits for our metabolism; therefore, I take it daily either in tablet, bath or cream form to ensure my magnesium levels are optimal.

Chapter 6: Unusual Diet

My Brief Dietary Background

Throughout my life, I tried many diets. None of the diets or approaches I tried based on mainstream advice worked for me. They all left some havoc which I had to fill in a costly way.

Some of those diet regimes genuinely damaged my health. Let's take the fruitarian diet as an example. I followed a fruitarian diet for few months. Unfortunately, it caused me to lose one of my teeth in the third month. I was only 28 years old. Even though it felt great in the beginning, after a few months just eating fruits was totally dangerous. Even though it was energising, I learnt that it was not a sustainable diet hence gave up after three months.

Then I tried a vegetarian diet, thinking that it was touted as the healthiest diet during that time. It was another big mistake for me. With all due respect to vegetarian friends, it was one of the worst diets on my health. I learnt that my genetic makeup does not support being vegetarian. As soon as I started a bit of meat, I started feeling better, and my health turned to average. I was still not satisfied with my overall performance.

Then I heard some commercial diets where they deliver food to your home. The amount of food is small, as their diet is based on portion control. I was starving all night, and hunger feelings were driving me crazy. Several times at night I was visiting the fridge but forcing my willpower to overcome the hunger feelings. It was the wrong choice. Yes, this diet worked a bit at helping me lose a few kilos, but it did not do anything worth mentioning here.

Discovering Unusual Diet

Why would I call this "unusual diet"? My reason is that the diet I will mention is not mainstream, and I believe that it has perceived side effects such as causing high cholesterol and hence is potentially linked to cardiovascular risks.

It is also [hypothetically] associated with cancer. The claims were only based on epidemiological studies. For example, I did not find any scientific study on just eating meat causing cancer.

I used to believe these perceptions floating in the media, several sources on the Internet and even some publications. However, when I started to review the medical and nutrition literature, there was hardly any evidence for these claims. With my personally acquired new knowledge, my confidence in transitioning to this diet became very easy.

My aim here is not to keep aside a new type of diet or blame other diets but to reveal how this unusual diet became beneficial for me. It is important to highlight that this diet made one of the most significant impacts on my health for improving my overall performance. Let me briefly explain this journey and how it happened.

The transition from Keto to Carnivore

After trying all other diets I mentioned earlier, it was serendipitous to come across with the Ketogenic, aka Keto, diet. The most significant contribution of the Keto diet for me is that it helped me become fat-adapted.

Several years I tried Keto and enjoyed it immensely. I never felt hungry or moody on this diet. Having an average of 1.5 nmol ketone levels floating in my bloodstream, I not only felt clear in my thinking but also my inflammation symptoms were considerably reduced.

As the Keto diet made me fat-adapted, I felt naturally ready to try the Carnivore diet. During that time (over five years ago) I did not know the name Carnivore, as it only appeared two years ago in the media, but I called it an all animal-based diet excluding dairy and eggs—in other words, an all-meat diet.

I removed the plants (vegetables and fruits) from my Keto diet. However, my fat intake was still high, but the source was only animal fat. When I was following the Keto diet, I used to drink a few spoons of olive oil every day and eat several spoons of butter.

Embracing Carnivore Diet

Moving from Keto to carnivore was very easy and effortless. The main change was cutting the plant sources from my diet. This included plant fats such as olive oil, nut oils and so on.

In the beginning, I was eating eggs and dairy in butter and kefir format. I used to love drinking homemade kefir. One day, I decided to remove eggs and dairy as well as my favourite kefir too. It was hard to give up kefir. I believed in its health benefits religiously but later experientially learned that it was not for my genetic makeup, so I sadly said goodbye to my beloved kefir.

Removing plants, dairy and eggs left me with only meat sources to survive and thrive. Let me explain what I eat on this unusual diet to survive and thrive.

I eat 100% animal meat, animal organs, animal fat and animal bones. That's it! My main diet includes mainly meat, bone, fat and organs from cows and sheep.

In addition, I eat fish and seafood three times a week. I learnt how to create a variety of dishes by using a combination of these food types. Like many others, I thought it might be boring, but it was more than I expected.

The main organs I include in my diet are liver, brain, kidneys, heart and bone marrow. Eating these organs helped me get all the essential minerals and vitamins which may be lacking in the muscle meat.

Recently I am pleased that some leading doctors on the Internet support eating organ meats. For example, one of my favourite doctors online (Dr Paul Saladino) calls this diet "eat[ing] an animal from nose to tail". I found his messages about a carnivore diet on the Internet potent and an excellent confirmation of my unusual diet.

I am so glad that there is a name for my unusual diet now and many people are trying it and gaining benefits from it. It is called the Carnivore diet. I like inspiring videos from Dr Sean Baker on YouTube, a talking the talk and walking the walk type of person I immensely respect. I was also impressed by Mikayla Patterson's and Amber O'Hearn's transformations, which I can closely relate to. I also want to mention amazing organ meat dishes and their importance to our health presented by Frank Tufano.

In addition to meat, I boil cow or lamb bones in the slow cooker for 24 hours and drink five to eight cups of bone broth every day. Drinking homemade bone broth every day provides several health benefits. The significant benefits are improving my digestion and sleep quality due to balancing my glycine content. I seemed to be lacking glycine in my previous diets, even in the Keto diet.

Boiling bones for 24 hours in the slow cooker also makes the bones very soft and crushable. I put the soft bones in a food processor like Nutri Bullet, which turns them into tiny pieces like flour. Crushed bones provide my daily natural calcium intake.

Adding crushed bones to a bone broth soup also makes it creamy and delicious when processed in a Nutri Bullet. Alternatively, I sometimes add a spoon of bone meal powder, which can be purchased from a health shop, if I run out of soft bones at home.

Fish and Seafood

I eat fish three to five times a week. The main fish I eat is wild cut salmon. Occasionally, I eat other fish such as mackerel and sardines.

My primary sources of seafood are prawns. Prawns are low-calorie food but provide complete high protein when I want to increase my protein intake on the fish and seafood days.

Despite my belief in the quality and comprehensiveness of this diet, I still have a few supplements. One essential supplement I have, especially on the days I do not eat fish, is a few fish or krill oil tablets. I know the critical benefits of omega 3 fatty acids on our brain and in reducing inflammation in our bodies.

What do I refrain from in this diet?

Even though there is hype on benefits of bacon as a carnivore meal, I do not eat any processed meat. Some people love it as it can be delicious.

I am also meticulous not to overcook or burn meat, as the side effects of overcooked or burnt meat are well documented. I usually cook my meat in an electric oven for 15-20 minutes.

Apart from harmful effects, overcooked meat or burnt barbecued meat is a turn off for me. My favourite cooking method is raw to medium, especially for steaks and salmon in an oven.

As mentioned earlier in my elimination diet regimen, I also don't eat any plant foods, eggs, and dairy.

Benefits from the Carnivore Diet

Over the past five years, just eating meat, organ meat, fish and prawns helped me feel like the best version of myself. Never has any diet made this much difference in my life; therefore, I am determined to continue it until I notice any negative implications. So far, I haven't experienced any adverse effects.

In summary, the key benefits of the Carnivore diet for me are digestive comfort, mental clarity, reduced-fat percentage, increased lean muscle mass, reduced inflammation, and reduced pain in muscles, joints and ligaments. In terms of digestive comfort, the most significant contributor was losing bloating. It is great to have a flat stomach.

Based on the benefits and transformational changes in my health, I have no intention of adding plants, dairy or eggs as long as I can keep this version of myself making me happy, joyful and satisfied.

Any Side Effects of the Carnivore Diet

Overall, I did not experience any side effects so far over the last five years. However, one minor point I work on is to address any potential excessive urea in the blood, which may be caused by excessive protein intake every now and then.

As I usually eat fatty meat and organ meats, it is not common for me to over-consume protein. My body knows when to stop as far as protein is concerned. It creates noticeable satiety. As imposed by my parents in my childhood, I usually don't leave any food on my plate. In this diet, ironically, there were times I had to stop and leave some of my favourite rib-eye steaks due to reaching satiety before finishing my meal. I don't throw out my leftover rib-eye, as it is costly in Australia. I eat it at my next meal.

However, as a precaution, I add three grams of citrulline malate to my water if I think I have overdosed on protein. Citrulline is an amino acid component of the urea cycle in the liver and helps to remove the urea. A few times, I tried ornithine and arginine, but they did not make any difference. I prefer citrulline, as the sour taste is appealing to me.

To verify, I tested for urea multiple times and noticed that urea in my blood was at a healthy level.

Digestive Enzymes

I love eating animal fats. My butcher thinks that I may die from cholesterol as he gives kilos of animal fat to me instead of tossing them into the rubbish bins. It is free because no one wants to buy animal fat due to fear of cholesterol. It is a controversial and significant topic, but I have no fear of cholesterol; instead, I embrace it. Every cell in our body needs it. Our body produces extra cholesterol when there is no food intake. It is a natural process. I learnt by testing that eating cholesterol may not possibly increase your cholesterol.

As mentioned earlier, I was doing the Ketogenic diet for many years. There were times I was overeating animal fats, especially when I had one meal a day plan. In one of these instances, a friend of mine who is a sports nutritionist introduced me to a digestive enzyme complex.

The supplement included vital enzymes such as Amylase, Protease, Lipase and other enzymatic ingredients like Betaine HCI and Ox Bile Extract. There were a few other enzymes too, but they were not major ones.

When I took a digestive enzyme supplement after a fatty meal, my indigestion symptoms disappeared. My stomach and gut were happy. I understand it is not essential for everyone, but it works well for me.

Since I mainly eat animal fat with some protein and almost no carbs, I only needed Protease and Lipase. Later I discovered pure Lipase in three different formats, such as Lipase, 1, 2 and 3. This well-formulated product made a real difference in improving my digestion.

I understand that the primary purpose of digestive enzymes is to break down food for energy. It was interesting to read from the nutrition- and diet-related publications that digestive enzymes can decrease inflammation, reduce symptoms of IBS, and even ease arthritis pain.

Salt

I didn't know how important salt was for our body, especially when I was in ketosis. Learning about the importance of salt and increasing my salt intake was a lifesaver for me. Salt helped me to overcome my keto flu and become fat-adapted in a very short time.

After increasing my salt intake, some muscular pain, especially in the early mornings, after 12 hours of fasting, disappeared.

Minor headaches disappeared after sipping a glass of saltwater with one teaspoon of Himalayan Pink Salt, Sea Salt or Redmond Real Salt.

I learnt to take salt after perspiring, especially in the sauna or after intensive cardio or weight training. It is a habit for me to carry salt in my emergency bag.

My blood pressure is normal, at the low end. For any reason, whenever my blood pressure goes down, I drink a glass of saltwater and it helps to turn my blood pressure back to normal.

Activated Charcoal

Charcoal is a miraculous ingredient in my diet. I take it once a week or occasionally when there is any stomach or gut upset. Nowadays, it rarely happens to me.

The key reason for taking activated charcoal once a week is to remove toxic minerals from my gut. As I eat fish at least three times a week, it is my belief that my body is exposed to some amount of mercury.

Since I take activated charcoal once a week two hours after the main meal, my digestion has improved a lot. It also helped improve my skin. I think that it may be due to the cleansing properties of activated charcoal.

Based on reviewed publications, my understanding is that activated charcoal traps toxins in the gut and prevents absorption of these toxins. The mechanism for this is that since activated charcoal is negatively charged, it attracts positively charged molecules like toxins. Then it helps these toxins to be removed from the body via faeces.

The caution is to take activated charcoal two hours after meals so that it does not interfere with digestion. Using it once a week provides the optimal solution to me. Taking it every day can be harmful, as it may also reduce other useful minerals in the gut.

Chapter 7: Effective Supplements

I use some supplements to boost my performance. These well-proven supplements added value to my wellbeing; hence, I added them as contributing factors to my transformation.

I would like to share these beneficial supplements here with you. Some of these supplements can sound controversial to some people, but I used them always with some scientific backing from prominent studies and discussions with my mentors, who also tried them safely.

These are not recommendations. The reason I pointed them out here is that these supplements truly helped me. They may not be as helpful to others. It is a reasonable practice that everyone does their own research, tries them based on their personal needs and circumstances, and of course, discusses with their trusted advisors, then takes full responsibility for the pros and cons.

Caffeine

Even though I love coffee and tea dearly, they upset my stomach; therefore, I cannot drink them. It is very disappointing to miss the smell and taste of freshly brewed coffee and some special tea such as Earl Grey. I cannot even enjoy herbal teas nowadays, as they upset my stomach too. For some reason, my body perceives anything from plants as a foreign material. I am now grateful to be aware of this. For many years I did not know about this intolerance, and with strong external influence on the benefits of plants, I suffered intensely.

Despite refraining from plants, caffeine is essential to

me for various reasons. Whoever says what about caffeine, for many years nothing has been as effective as caffeine for my cognitive boost and nothing helped me better to get rid of my occasional mild depression without any noticeable side effects. It is beyond dependence, as multiple times I gave up and tried to survive without caffeine and replaced it with other so-called 'adaptogenic supplements' like ginseng, ashwagandha, turmeric and so on. They all made me feel worse, with many unbearable side effects, including ongoing bloating.

My caffeine use is very specific, controlled and monitored. It is not a habitual act anymore. It is a tool to be used when required. I only use caffeine tablets in the mornings with careful timing and in exact doses. It is evident that if caffeine is taken afternoons for most people, it can cause sleep disturbances. This is true for me too.

Therefore, I take a 200 mg caffeine tablet on the days when I need to go to work or the gym early. The caffeine tablets I use do not cause any stomach upset as opposed to coffee, tea or caffeinated drinks. In addition, I can be sure about the exact amount of caffeine intake with tablets, as this knowledge was not possible with drinking coffee or tea. Depending on the quality of coffee or tea, the dose may be very different.

I know some of you will not approve this hack due to its controversial nature but sincerely, using caffeine tablets at certain times improved my life quality when taken with responsible dosing and timing. It still helps me immensely when I take it before noon when needed; therefore, I am sharing this small hack here with confidence and no shame.

Nicotine

Here is another controversial supplement, but please

keep reading to understand this madness behind my order. I am not a smoker and not definitely recommend anyone to smoke. It is a harmful habit which was scientifically proven.

The first time I heard about the benefits of nicotine on the human cognitive process was when I was undertaking my doctoral degree in the mid-90s. It was communicated to us by one of our Cognitive Science lectures in an elegant way. We were all surprised by the science behind the benefits of nicotine, and some smokers were nodding with triumph. However, it had nothing to do with smoking.

Since then there are some further studies conducted on short term benefits of pure nicotine, especially on memory, in a very low dose, such as implemented in a patch or via chewing a piece of gum. It was particularly pointed out that nicotine should come from patch, gum, or lozenges but not cigarettes as the smoke of cigarettes was proven to hold multiple toxic agents harmful to one's health.

I don't smoke but tried nicotine gums occasionally during difficult exams at my postgraduate studies and complex problem-solving sessions at work. It was helpful to reduce my stress and anxiety and keep my motivation as far as I needed.

Fortunately, I did not experience any side effects except some bitter taste of the gum. One time, I tried a patch, but it made the patching point very itchy for me, so I did not continue using it again.

However, since there are no long-term studies established on the effects of supplemental pure nicotine yet, I am a little hesitant making this as a usual supplement for myself, so I rarely use it — only when I really need it.

N-Acetyl-Tyrosine

Tyrosine is an amino acid which we normally get from

our protein intake. My understanding is that this amino acid is used in our body to produce hormones such as epinephrine, noradrenaline, and dopamine.

I specifically use this version of tyrosine (N-Acetyl-Tyrosine) as an effective supplement to increase my mental alertness when needed. This version has an additional active compound called "acetic acid" attached to it. Adding acetic acid to tyrosine increases bioavailability and absorption when we digest it.

Even though some side effects such as nausea are mentioned in the literature, I personally did not notice any side effect by having 350 mg intake in a fasted state, for occasional use, usually in the mornings. When I combine this supplement with a half caffeine tablet (100 mg), it can be even more effective for my alertness and motivation on my challenging mornings.

N-Acetyl-Cysteine

Cysteine is another amino acid. It is not a drug or medication. The version of cysteine I use is a supplemental form called N-Acetyl-Cysteine (NAC).

My main reason for using this supplement daily is to help the natural creation of glutathione in my body. As is well documented in medical literature, glutathione is the master antioxidant in our body. NAC is a co-factor for the creation of glutathione. I occasionally take 600 mg of this supplement.

Even though there is a direct glutathione boosting supplement, it is not recommended by the medical professionals as it may adversely impact the body's natural production of this critical antioxidant. Therefore, NAC is considered a viable alternative.

As a well-studied supplement, I learnt many other

benefits of NAC. For example, in summary, NAC can help the detoxification process in the body, can regulate glutamate levels in our brain, can reduce symptoms of some psychiatric disorders and hence can reduce addictive behaviour.

In addition, NAC can relieve symptoms of respiratory conditions, can decrease inflammation in fat tissue, can reduce insulin resistance, and can increase immune function. To me, it is a miracle supplement. I had no noticeable side effects after occasional use of it, such as once or twice a week, around 600 mg, over the last five years.

Alpha Lipoic Acid

As an organic compound, Alpha Lipoic Acid can be found in all human cells, inside the mitochondria. It is not only a profound antioxidant but also as suggested by recent research studies; it can play a role in weight management and support of other metabolic activities in the body.

My reason to include Alpha Lipoic Acid as an occasional supplement to my diet is the recycling capability of vitamin C and vitamin E. I don't supplement vitamins C and E.

Additional benefits of Alpha Lipoic Acid that I learned are the ability to slow skin aging, improve nerve function, lower blood sugar levels, and reduce inflammation.

It was recommended to me by many bio-hackers who have advanced degrees or vast experience in various medical fields. Even though some side effects such as getting nauseated are documented, I did not experience any noticeable side effects by taking 600 mg occasionally, like once or twice a week, over the last five years.

NADH

NADH stands for Nicotinamide Adenine Dinucleotide.

NADH is the active coenzyme form of vitamin B3. It naturally occurs in the body and plays an important role in the energy production of every human cell.

Low NADH is linked to several metabolic problems in the body, such as weight gain, chronic fatigue syndrome, and cardiovascular problems.

Optimised NADH is critical for DNA repair, improved metabolism, and overall healthy cellular function. Our energy powerhouse, Mitochondria, gets its electrons from NADH.

We can increase NADH with a better diet, intense exercise, use of dry sauna, and other healthy practices. However, after reading the recent research documenting the effects of low and optimised NADH levels, I decided to supplement.

The risks and side effects are also reasonable to me. One key point I learnt is using NADH with a supplement called TMG (trimethylglycine) to address potential methylation issues.

After I started using NADH supplement in 10 mg occasionally, once or twice a week, over the last three years, I felt improved mental clarity, more alertness, better concentration on my daily activities, and experienced reduced fatigue, especially in the afternoons.

I am still not one hundred per cent sure I will continue with NADH as a supplement, but the recent studies for its effect on brain activities sound breathtaking. Therefore, I am closely watching the progress for NADH research and can decide to proceed based on the results.

Chapter 8: Daily Health Focus

Overall Inflammation Awareness

Inflammation is inevitable in our bodies. It is a natural healing process. However, there are times it can be excessive and cause a myriad of problems for our health. Almost every disease is associated with chronic inflammation.

My body was producing excessive inflammation for some unknown reason. I suffered for many years with no proper diagnosis. After further investigations by medical specialists, the main culprit seemed to be rheumatoid arthritis. For many years, it was not detected and caused me immense suffering.

During those years, I was not aware of the importance of inflammation in our health. I had not even considered it as a life-changing factor. I thought it was just a condition my body had and accepted it blindly and with a kind of victim mentality. One of my specialists was saying there was no cure for it so I must be on Voltaren tablets for a lifetime, and if symptoms increase, they might have considered regular injections to reduce my inflammation.

I was so naïve to have so much trust in medical professionals and institutions in those days. This is a big regret for having such a passive attitude. After discovering a self-managed healing approach, as mentioned in this book, I promised myself never to accept mainstream medical advice again without thoroughly questioning the rationale and looking for alternatives.

My view on inflammation totally changed after witnessing some inflammatory conditions, such as an autoimmune disease in my beloved ones. I understood the critical significance of inflammation in our lives. My father died at a relatively young age because of inflammatory autoimmune disease, even though he was very healthy from every other aspect and followed the mainstream advice religiously. As he followed a heavily plant-based diet, refraining from red meat for fear of perceptive cancer and cardiovascular diseases, his vitamin B12 levels were found to be extremely low and sadly it was only detected after the damage occurred to his motor neurons.

This poignant suffering motivated me to further investigate the nature and implications of inflammation in our lives. My findings were an eye-opener for me that most of the diseases were linked to or associated with inflammation in the medical literature. Ironically, I found that intolerance to the so-called healthiest plants was establishing some root causes of it in my condition.

It is essential to point out that the emphasis of implications on health was on the chronic inflammation, the type of inflammation which stays in the body for an extended period of time, not the short term, acute inflammation which is a natural healing necessity.

It was clear that acute inflammation is even considered healthy because the body attempts to fix an underlying issue such as a cut or injury. Acute inflammation is a built-in healing mechanism in the human body, so I embrace it, especially after intense gym sessions.

Once I learned about the impact of inflammation, especially the side effects of chronic inflammation on our health, I started learning how to address the root causes of inflammation and consequently reduce those symptoms.

Several of the previously mentioned hacks in this book helped in dealing with my inflammatory conditions in an effective way. For example, simply changing my diet to zero carbs, tapping into my body fat as a primary energy source, and producing ketones naturally made a tremendously favourable impact on my inflammation.

As soon as my body was producing ketones around 1.5 nmol, most of the painful feelings disappeared from my body. My family doctor couldn't believe in the progress of my inflammation markers in my blood test, and he even requested further tests. It was my fault I didn't disclose my zero-carb diet to my doctor, as he did not like it once I asked him about his opinion. Despite his disapproval, I adapted a zero-carb diet to improve my health by taking personal responsibility.

My doctor requested several blood markers for inflammation. For example, I still regularly check my CRP (C-reactive Protein), ESR (Erythrocyte Sedimentation Rate) and PV (Plasma Viscosity) once every six months.

The most prominent causes of inflammation in my case were evident of having excessive carbs such as slices of bread, pasta, rice, potato and so-called healthy fruit juice in my previous diets. The evil impact was coupled with inefficient stress management techniques, including broken sleep patterns.

In addition to changing my diet, introducing stress management tools such as dry sauna, baths with Epsom salts, undertaking joyful exercises and improving my sleep quality made excellent contributions to reducing chronic inflammation in my body. With reduced inflammation, I feel younger, happier and healthier.

Blood Monitoring

For many years I was on high carb diets, eating lots of

bread, rice, and potatoes, and drinking excessive freshly squeezed fruit juices. I thought fruit juice was the healthiest drink. After each meal and drinking fruit juice, I always felt lethargic, especially in the afternoons.

I thought it was a reasonable human condition to be lethargic in the afternoons. However, sometimes when I saw very energetic people, full of beans all the time, around me, I was thinking that they were highly caffeinated or taking energizing drugs, or genetically gifted. In hindsight, this was poor judgement.

When I learnt about the importance of blood sugar fluctuations on our moods, energy levels and overall mental health, I wanted to check my blood sugar levels. During that time, one enticing fact was that our bloodstream could only get around one teaspoon of sugar at a time, whereas I was getting many spoonfuls of sugar from multiple food sources and fruit juices, including sugared coffee and tea, which were my regular drinks on those days. How ignorant and misinformed I was! Ironically, my caretaking doctors never pointed out that my poor diet was source of my suffering.

With my curiosity, one day, I found an affordable blood glucose monitoring device from eBay and purchased glucose test strips from the pharmacy. The pharmacist was interrogating me whether I was diabetic, as the cost of private purchase was very high. It took a while to convince her that I might be prediabetic; therefore, I needed to check my blood sugar to ensure it was within acceptable ranges daily. She was insisting I should purchase it through the Medicare system due to its prohibitive cost. When it comes to my health, especially bio-hacking myself safely, cost is not an issue at all.

It was astonishing to see my blood sugar was going high after the main meals. Fruit juices were skyrocketing it. I wondered how fruit juice was recommended to kids and adults, especially for breakfast. My elevated blood sugar took four hours to settle into a healthy range.

This simple test motivated me to reduce my carbs and increase my protein and fat intake. Initially, in a week or so, I felt a bit lethargic due to keto flu, but in the second week my energy level boosted high. I suddenly started feeling fantastic. I welcomed a new version of myself with a simple hack!

With this minor yet incredible improvement in my overall health, I started searching further to understand low carb, high-fat diets. I came across the Ketogenic diet, which was a fantastic transformation for my overall health, both physically and mentally. Even though I heard many negative aspects of the Ketogenic diet, with lots of scary notions, they did not mean anything to me because it was an ideal diet for my body.

Every negative aspect of the Ketogenic diet faded away, as none of those undesirable conditions happened to me. Everything was just the opposite. I provide more information about my dietary background in the chapter on an unusual diet in this book.

With this enthusiasm, I started testing my blood sugar and ketone levels every day, a few times a day, keeping a record of them in a spreadsheet and creating data sets including my weight, belly size, fat percentage, muscle quality, sleep time, calorie intake, blood pressure, amount of salts, and many more daily measures. I practised my data architecture skills in monitoring my health in detail.

Seeing optimal blood sugar and elevated ketone levels much motivated me to keep these records religiously for several months. A few months later, I entirely became fat-adapted, and my terrible hunger feelings disappeared. My energy level was similar to when I was a teenager. In fact, at 50+ years old, I was wearing my jeans bought at the age of 18.

My thinking became more explicit and my mood was always on the positive and optimistic side. My family members, friends and colleagues were teasing me whether I undertook antiaging therapies like Botox or other body improvement methods.

With this energy and enthusiasm, I increased my exercise times, both aerobic and anaerobic (cardio and weight training formats). Exercise helped even further optimise my blood sugar levels and increase my ketone levels. Being in high ketosis at most times made me feel almost euphoric. No, I did not lose any muscles!

My problem solving, attention, mental flexibility, agility, and memory skills also improved. As mentioned in another section, I am subscribed to Lumosity and Elevate to measure my mental skills such as memory, attention, problem solving, flexibility and agility. My daily practices of mind games dramatically showed improvement.

A simple blood monitoring curiosity opened new ways for my diet, physical exercise regimen and mental efforts. I still test my blood glucose and ketone levels but not as frequently as I used to in the first year. My body is so attuned that I even can guess my blood glucose and ketone levels by observing my daily behaviour.

Then I also learnt that there are many other blood tests monitoring for other aspects of our health. Our family doctors conduct only minimal blood tests, and like any average citizen, I thought they were adequate to learn about our health profile. It was another mistake to believe mainstream claims on unnecessary blood tests. They were unsubstantiated.

The next level for me was to take the specialist level tests. I was pleased to know that a specialist — for example, an endocrinologist — could conduct many hormonal tests to create a profile of the hormonal situation. As Medicare did not support, I paid specialist medical professionals to provide me insights through multiple essential blood tests. In my opinion, this was a good investment for my health. If I left my conditions to mainstream and Medicare, I could have died by now.

In addition, I learnt that there are many special blood tests that we can get done through online pathologies with no prescription. Some are sophisticated and expensive tests. They can provide useful insights into our health situation. In addition to blood tests, I even got my DNA tested online privately and obtained insightful findings. My family doctor said it was a waste of time. But it was worth the investment, as a few simple pointers really provided valuable lessons for me and validated a few suspicious situations about my genetic predisposition.

Dental Health

We all know about the importance of dental hygiene. In general, it can help prevent tooth decay, gum disease and even bad breath. Gum disease and associated inflammation are also linked to cardiovascular disease.

My understanding of the mechanism for gum disease leading to heart problems is the inflammation in the mouth also affects the inflammation of the arteries. This inflammation of the arteries can cause the development of atherosclerotic plaques. These types of plaques in the arteries can increase the risk of a heart attack or even cause a stroke.

With this knowledge, I learnt to pay more attention to my dental health. A straightforward measure was to increase brushing my teeth three times a day. I used to brush twice.

For many years I went to a dentist at least once a year. My dentists talked about the importance of tooth brushing and flossing. However, a few years ago, I came across interdental brushing, which made the most significant contribution to my dental hygiene.

The problem I found was that tooth brushing and flossing did not always clean between all the tooth grooves. Because of this limitation, harmful plaque and tartar can develop quickly in these hard-to-reach places of our dental systems.

I experienced that the solution to cleaning between the tooth grooves was using interdental brushes. They are specially shaped to reach into teeth grooves to remove debris and plaque. I understood that interdental brushing was the most effective solution in preventing bacterial colonization causing tooth decay.

In addition to interdental brushing, recently I also came across a new toothpaste including activated charcoal. I always use activated charcoal for other purposes but never used it for dental hygiene before. This specific toothpaste formulated with activated charcoal helped me remove the stains on my teeth more effectively.

Contrary to the advice of my dentists, I use natural mouth washing liquids between the brushing times to rejuvenate my mouth. With the introduction of natural mouth washing liquids, I even noticed more improvement in my dental health, but my dentists do not believe it. It is fine with me, as I respect their view but practice my proven tactics to experience the benefits. My health is not a dental discussion point. My true feelings and personal experiences drive my motivation.

Skin Health

Undeniably, the skin is the largest organ in our body; hence it requires a great deal of attention. Skin health is a broad topic. It touches many disciplines and lifestyle factors such as nutrition, exercise, sun exposure, cleaning, cooling, drying, moisturizing and so on.

I am mindful not to load your brains with lots of details on any of these things in this focused book. There are other publications dealing with those broad topics. However, one key point I want to emphasise here is the use of dry brushing.

I experience that dry brushing can stimulate the nervous system. It is enjoyable to use dry brushing on our itchy skin. I understand that it can help detoxify by increasing blood circulation in the skin. It can also unclog pores.

This small tool and the simple process made a big difference in my skin health. Whenever I feel itchy, I use dry brushing rather than scratching my skin with my nails. Scratching with nails can damage our skin. However, dry brushing really addresses the itching problem without any harsh impact on the skin.

In addition to dry brushing, regular moisturizing with sorbolene lotion or magnesium sulphate water solution and exfoliating with soft fibre are the most significant contributors to my skin health.

Dry Sauna

Dry sauna has been one of my best stress management tools by adding extra pleasure to my life. Apart from addressing my past inflammation issues, there are a few reasons that I enjoy a sauna so much.

It is well known that the heat in a dry sauna induces quickly noticeable physiological effects. More specifically, the heat can increase skin and core body temperature quickly. The quick increase in body temperature can also increase heart rate, skin blood flow, and cause perspiration rapidly.

The way I enjoy a sauna is taking it in a few small sessions between 15 to 20 minutes, depending on the temperature of the sauna. After 10 minutes, I can experience a lot of perspiration in many parts of my body, most substantial on the face. Then, I have a quick break, like five minutes outside. Then I try another 15 minutes, but after that I have a cold shower.

Having cold showers after an intense sauna session feels excellent. After the third or fourth session, depending on my time, I keep cooling down with cold showers. I can check from my smartwatch that most of the time, my pulse fluctuates up and down. For example, it reaches to 150 beats per second when inside the sauna after 15 minutes and drops back to 60 beats per second after having cold showers for five minutes outside the sauna.

An hour after the last sauna session, most of my stress disappears. I feel productive, both physically and mentally. The physical manifestation is relaxed muscles, joints, and ligaments. Any exercise-induced pain quickly melts away. Even my anxieties and worries go away.

There is a growing body of literature documenting many more benefits of dry saunas, such as improving cardiovascular health, removing toxins and improving the immune system, inducing deep sleep, reducing Alzheimer's risks, and even improving longevity by activating SIRT2 genes.

I haven't fully experienced all these benefits yet and am open-minded about them; however, I have certainly enjoyed the stress and pain management aspects of the sauna, and it has become a pleasant hobby and a regular transformational tool for me.

I am further stretching this to the point that maybe large innovative organisations such as Google, Apple and Pixar should add a dry sauna and accompanying cold shower facilities to their offices. This unusual investment can provide fantastic positive returns with improved employee health and wellbeing.

Body Fat & Lean Muscle Awareness

In addition to looking good and well-shaped, low body fat has multiple health benefits. Lean muscle mass is essential for all of us. A combination of lean muscle mass and low body fast is linked to increased hormonal stability, increased metabolism, increased flexibility in joints, tendons, ligaments, and increased bone density. These are desirable characteristics as we get older.

In addition to exercise, proper nutrition, sleep and rest, I strive to monitor my body fat and muscle quality. To this end, I go to an elite sports centre using Dexa Scan mainly for professional sportspeople such as soccer and cricket players and gymnasts. It is the gold standard to measure fat, muscle and bone mass accurately.

Due to demand and its scarcity, using Dexa Scan is an expensive practice. For example, I paid $180 for one session in Australia. My son was teasing me that learning two-digit numbers about my body on a piece of paper cost such a large amount of money. Dexa Scan sessions also require booking several weeks ahead, as they are not very common in some cities or countries.

To address the cost issue, my solution was to measure my body fat percentage and muscle quality via the use of a hand-held device called Skulp. It was around $100 to purchase online. It came from the USA. The device links to an app on the smartphone and the results are close to the Dexa Scan. I am impressed with the accuracy of the Skulp.

Simply monitoring my body fat and muscle quality by using Skulp once a month motivates me to keep my body fat lower and to strengthen my lean muscles. I can also see the historical values in the Skulp app on my smartphone.

Intermittent Fasting

Intermittent fasting was one of the best tools I used to improve my health from almost all aspects of my transformation. In summary, it helped me reduce my body fat, improve my lean muscle mass, and improve my mental sharpness.

The easiest way to implement intermittent fasting is by skipping breakfast. Despite the mainstream's unsubstantiated warnings, I learnt that breakfast was not the most important meal of the day. I did not have any breakfast for over ten years, and I felt better and better by practising this simple hack.

Some of my family members and colleagues were telling me that it was unhealthy not to have breakfast. I did not experience any side effects caused by intermittent fasting. With my unusual diet, it is even more effective and much more comfortable, as I am already fat-adapted. I rarely feel hungry. My hunger is not emotional, as it used to be when I was on high carb diets. Now if I am hungry, that means I am physically hungry, and my body needs to replenish, not to satisfy cravings. By the way, I never crave for any food any more.

To emphasise, using an intermittent fasting regimen, I experience no muscle loss, as I regularly measure them as pointed out in the previous section. The reason I highlight this here is that there are some rumours and baseless claims in the media about muscle loss risks associated with intermittent fasting. They are contrary to my experience; in fact, I gain better lean muscle on this regimen.

Mitochondria Awareness

Whenever I hear or read the term "Mitochondria", it

brings me the image of energy powerhouses of our cells. Mitochondria are organelles that create ATP (Adenosine Triphosphate) via cellular respiration by breaking nutrients and creating energy molecules for our cells.

It is essential to be aware of mitochondrial health. When our mitochondria are damaged or malfunctioning, our overall energy level and daily performance drop dramatically. We start feeling lethargic, tired, and lazy. It can be noticeable both mentally and physically.

Mitochondria is a well-researched topic. We know that our nutrition, exercise regimen, sleep habits, and resting habits have considerable impacts on the health of mitochondria. In addition, toxins have a negative impact on the proper functioning of mitochondria.

Even though genetics plays an important role, I learnt from literature and my mentors that most of the hacks I introduced in this book can have positive impact on mitochondria—for example, reducing stress, eliminating toxins from the body, decreasing fat, improving lean muscle mass, eating nutrient-dense food, exercise, sleep, rest, and dry saunas.

Doing Less, Achieving More

Doing less and achieving more is a principle I learned in the early 90s during my doctoral studies. One of our lecturers, who was also one of my supervisors, taught me to focus on important tasks to complete my doctorate. Due to the nature of doctoral studies, one can easily be distracted and digress to a myriad of other attractive ideas and diverse content not necessarily core to the fundamental idea being researched.

Each time when we met, my supervisor was asking what important tasks I planned to undertake on that day. He kept asking me about my priorities and wanted to review them and provide instant feedback. He emphasized that it was the key point to complete my studies on time and what he called "effortlessly".

With this approach, he was also helping me to reduce my stress. Focusing on only the things that genuinely matter reduces the unnecessary load I used to carry prior to meeting him. Since I love learning, I was quickly digressing to many different unrelated areas, and it was creating unnecessary stress for me.

This specific academic supervisor helped me understand the importance of 80/20 rule in making my priorities. I also learnt from him not to manage time but to manage my priorities. He was wisely echoing that time was not manageable. Learning to complete small tasks in a systematic priority order helped me to complete my research and write my thesis on time.

In addition, I applied to do less and to achieve more principle in my work. Applying this principle at work helped me to be a role model professional and leader in my field. This has been one of the most effective methods that helped me transform to a more satisfying life. I love doing less and achieving more.

Removing Clutter

It has been a great feeling to reduce clutter in my life. I pay particular attention daily to remove unnecessary things at home and in the workplace.

Whenever I look at an object in my home, my first couple of questions are "do I really need this, or can I do without this object"? This simple questioning habit helps me to have an uncluttered lifestyle.

As the years go by, I have adopted the importance of

the less is more principle and reaped the benefits of it. Therefore, my points in this book are concise and unelaborated as opposed to other books on similar topics.

I don't like adding many case studies of annoying fictitious people, unnecessary hypothetical situations, and excessive historical information. Cutting the clutter in verbal and written communication by being direct and to the point is the communication strategy that works best for me.

Taking Full Responsibility

The best lesson I learnt in my childhood from my parents was taking full responsibility for everything I did in my life. This principle has been one of the most critical transformational factors in every aspect of my life.

Using this principle helped me not to blame anyone for anything. Blaming is the default mode for the brain. It is effortless to blame someone or something for the undesirable outcomes we experience. It is challenging to take full responsibility, especially in stressful situations.

I learnt young that whenever my brain goes to the blame mode for anything for any reason, I must make a special effort to stop myself and find a gratitude point, even in the most challenging situations.

I also experienced that in hindsight, most of the problematic points and undesirable situations turned into blessings in disguise. This mindset helped me to be more grateful and less whiny.

The content of this whole book clearly reflects the importance of taking full responsibility for my life. It is important to me that I like testing controversial approaches by taking a personal risk and not by blaming the publications or anyone who recommended them to me when they don't work.

Instead of blaming an individual, a publication or

institution, such as in my case, poor mainstream medical advice at an earlier age, I chose to change my path and take responsibility for my own health. I still respect my family doctors, specialist doctors, or hospitals but I always do my own research for my health to make the final decision based on informed choices.

It is important to point once more, I don't recommend anything to anyone, but instead, I love sharing my experiences and narrate them naturally, without hype or bias. Even though sharing personal facts may put me in a vulnerable situation, they are still worth sharing. There is the possibility that some people may try to take advantage of one's vulnerability. Since I am aware of the risks, it is not a problem to share my experiences most of the time.

Acting Now

The importance of now is well known and well documented in interdisciplinary studies. There are special emphases of "now" on business, commerce, psychology, religion, economy, medicine, engineering, art and other disciplines.

Taking immediate action for the things that genuinely matter became second nature to me. This principle relates to anything and at any time for things requiring completion. I do not like procrastinating. As soon as I see my brain go to the default procrastination mode, I try to have a friendly conversation with my brain and kindly ask it to turn to action orientation. Most of the time, my trained brain obeys nicely and we become friends again.

From earlier days, it was one of the most useful things to learn how to stop procrastinating in my life. A straightforward implementation of this for me is that if I believe the task at hand can be done in a few minutes, I never leave it to a later time.

However, if a task requires further analysis and thinking, then I plan an appropriate time to undertake it and take action based on the plan and the priority set for the task. If the task cannot be completed at a specific time, the best approach is to deconstruct the task to smaller chunks and tackle them in priority order for each identified component.

Dealing with smaller tasks and completing high priority ones earlier can motivate us. Tasting the success of the completion of small tasks, I noticed that my brain serves me better, with more enthusiasm instead of withdrawal or procrastination symptoms.

It is a personal inspiration for me to focus on now and on the specific (prioritized) tasks at hand. This awareness helped me move from my comfort zone. I love my stretch zone. Being in the stretch zone helps me create my future by taking timely action and personal responsibility for my actions.

Being an action-oriented person helped me to be more courageous, despite my fears, in scary situations. In fact, taking timely action has been the only tool to help me overcome my fears. Timely actions equal courage. Delayed actions can intensify fear and may even paralyse us by demanding we stay passive in the comfort zone.

Authoring this book was one of the actions I put off despite some initial anxiety at sharing my personal experience publicly. However, despite the initial concern, the belief that my experience may help other people and provide some insights to those who need some examples from real life encouraged me to proceed and take action. My fear disappeared when I was halfway through authoring this book. I wrote this book in my stretch zone and hope you read it in your stretch zone as well. Reading these transformational points can make better sense in the stretch zone. If you read this book in default mode and comfort zone, most of these points will look very difficult.

In addition, I'd love to get feedback and learn from my readers' experience related to these items that worked for my desired transformation. Who knows? Perhaps I can learn more from your experience for transforming to better experiences. You may validate my trials as positive or negative based on your own experience. I can be contacted via LinkedIn, which is my primary social media site. I also engaged in Goodreads, interacting with many readers and authors. I hope to converse with you in my other books too.

Convenient Learning

Learning is one of my strongest desires and continuous practice in my life. In the past, I used to read many books, especially as a recreational activity. Every point in this book is a learnt activity. I even wrote a comprehensive thesis about learning in technical and scientific settings. As the topic is too broad, I do not want to go into any detail about learning in this book.

My point is related to reading. Let me explain. Reading from a book or an electronic device requires certain conditions and prerequisites, such as full attention and a comfortable and quiet location. However, with the help of technology, I extended my reading to using Audible publications. This became a strong point for me; hence I wanted to share it with you too.

In order to listen to some essential publications on the go, I used to purchase expensive tapes, CDs and DVDs. They had their own limitations. However, the audio streaming services like Audible are the most convenient to listen and learn almost anywhere with any device.

I found the Audible subscription model very useful to

speed up my learning. This subscription is economical and effective to access many books in audible format. Having said that, I still enjoy reading books when it is possible.

Chapter 9: Conclusion

In this concise book, I provided a brief narration of essential transformational items in my life. Most of them were on a trial and error basis and only became second nature after experiencing difficulties in my life.

Instead of being a victim of the established systems, I chose to learn based on experience by piggybacking my scientific background and leveraging the experience of my mentors and those brave people who shared their personal experiences in various media.

The primary message of this book is reinventing myself. For many years, I made a conscious effort to reinvent myself to newer versions. Let me briefly disclose why I keep reinventing myself.

Reinventing Myself

People around me pose questions like why I keep trying new hacks all the time and take a considerable amount of risk in my life. My simple answer is to reach the best version of myself by reinventing myself.

As I find new meanings in my life, the changes I plan become naturally inevitable. We know that everything in life keeps changing, so we need to adapt to the constant change. Instead of random or ad hoc changes, I prefer planned changes. Creating planned changes gives a delightful sense of control over my destiny.

Considering the limits of my mind and body, their capacity at a given time, I try to increase the physical and mental load incrementally. As I learn and try new things, each increment causes some positive change and helps me reinvent new versions of myself. Over the last decade, I experienced multiple versions of myself and immensely enjoyed each version.

Reinvention is an ongoing process for me, and I am assuming for you too. Reinvention occurs in my occupation, hobbies, relationships, creativity, physical posture, flexibility, speed, strength, sleep quality, stress tolerance, physical endurance, communications, and several other life aspects.

Understanding the message of my feelings and my emotions, recurring thought patterns, aligned with controlled logic, help me migrate from a comfort zone to a well-designed and transformed stretch zone.

I keep looking inside out and outside in to understand what touches me at what level, what inspires me, and what influences me. Learning more and knowing more about myself each day through trial and error can also help me to re-create my newer versions.

All the items mentioned in this book helped me from various angles to transform into newer versions of myself as I set them to achieve my desired goals in my growth plan and life satisfaction strategy.

It was an honour and pleasure to share my modest insights with you. I hope to learn your insights and how you reinvent yourself. You can follow me on Amazon for further updates on this book and my other books that may be an interest to you. The link to my author page on Amazon is amazon.com/author/drmehmetyildiz

Other Books By This Author

A Modern Enterprise Architecture Approach Empowered with Mobility, Cloud, IoT & Big Data

Modernise and transform the enterprise with pragmatic architecture, powerful technologies, innovative agility, and fusion

I authored this book to provide essential guidance, compelling ideas, and unique ways to Enterprise Architects so that they can successfully perform complex enterprise modernisation initiatives transforming from chaos to coherence. This is not an ordinary theory book describing Enterprise Architecture in detail. There are myriad of books on the market and in libraries discussing details of enterprise architecture.

As a practicing Senior Enterprise Architect myself, I read hundreds of those books and articles to learn different views. They have been valuable to me to establish my foundations in the earlier phase of my profession. However, what is missing now is a concise guidance book showing Enterprise Architects the novel approaches, insights from the real-life experience and experimentations, and pointing out the differentiating technologies for enterprise modernisation. If only there were such a guide when I started engaging in modernisation and transformation programs.

The biggest lesson learned is the business outcome of the enterprise modernisation. What genuinely matters for business is the return on investment of the enterprise architecture and its monetising capabilities. The rest is the theory because nowadays sponsoring executives, due to economic climate, have no interest, attention, or tolerance for non-profitable ventures. I am sorry for disappointing some idealistic Enterprise Architects, but with due respect, it is the reality, and we cannot change it. This book deals with reality rather than theoretical perfection. Anyone against this view on this climate must be coming from another planet.

In this concise, uncluttered and easy-to-read book, I attempt to show the significant pain points and valuable considerations for enterprise modernisation using a structured approach. The architectural rigour is still essential. We cannot compromise the rigour aiming to the quality of products and services as a target outcome. However, there must be a delicate balance among architectural rigour, business value, and speed to market. I applied this pragmatic approach to multiple substantial transformation initiatives and complex modernisations programs. The key point is using an incrementally progressing iterative approach to every aspect of modernisation initiatives, including people, processes, tools, and technologies as a whole.

Starting with a high-level view of enterprise architecture to set the context, I provided a dozen of distinct chapters to point out and elaborate on the factors which can make a real difference in dealing with complexity and producing excellent modernisation initiatives. As eminent leaders, Enterprise Architects are the critical talents who can undertake this massive mission using their people and technology skills, in addition to many critical attributes such as calm and composed approach. They are architects, not firefighters. I have full confidence that this book can provide valuable insights and aha moments for these talented architects to tackle this enormous mission turning chaos to coherence.

Architecting secure, agile, economic, highly available, well-performing IoT ecosystems

The focus of this book is to provide IoT solution architects with practical guidance and a unique perspective. Solution architects working in IoT ecosystems have an unprecedented level of responsibility at work; therefore, dealing with IoT ecosystems can be daunting.

As an experienced practitioner of this topic, I understand the challenges faced by the IoT solution architects. In this book, I have reflected upon my insights based on my solution architecture experience spread across three decades. In addition, this book can also guide other architects and designers who want to learn the architectural aspects of IoT and understand the key challenges and practical resolutions in IoT solution architectures. Each chapter focuses on the key aspects that form the framing scope for this book; namely, security, availability, performance, agility, and cost-effectiveness.

In this book, I have also provided useful definitions, a brief practical background on IoT and a guiding chapter on solution architecture development. The content is mainly practical; hence, it can be applied or be a supplemental input to the architectural projects at hand.

Transform enterprise with technical excellence, innovation, simplicity, agility, fusion, and collaboration

The primary purpose of this book is to provide valuable insights for digital transformational leadership empowered by technical excellence by using a pragmatic five-pillar framework. This empowering framework aims to help the reader understand the common characteristics of technical and technology leaders in a structured way.

Even though there are different types of leaders in broad-spectrum engaging in digital transformations, in this book, we only concentrate on excellent technical and technology leaders having digital transformation goals to deal with technological disruptions and robust capabilities to create new revenue streams. No matter whether these leaders may hold formal executive titles or just domain specialist titles, they demonstrate vital characteristics of excellent technical leadership capabilities enabling them to lead complex and complicated digital transformation initiatives.

The primary reason we need to understand technical excellence and required capabilities for digital transformational leadership in a structured context is to model their attributes and transfer the well-known characteristics to the aspiring leaders and the next generations. We can transfer our understanding of these capabilities at an individual level and apply them to our day to day activities. We can even turn them into useful habits to excel in our professional goals. Alternatively, we can pass this information to other people that we are responsible for, such as our teenagers aiming for digital leadership roles, tertiary students, mentees, and colleagues.

We attempt to define the roles of strategic technical and

technology leaders using a specific framework, based on innovation, simplicity, agility, collaboration, fusion and technical excellence. This framework offers a common understanding of the critical factors of the leader. The structured analysis presented in this book can be valuable to understand the contribution of technical leaders clearly.

Admittedly, this book has a bias towards the positive attributes of excellent leaders on purpose. The compelling reason for this bias is to focus on the positive aspects and describe these attributes concisely in an adequate amount to grasp the topic so that these positive attributes can be reused and modelled by the aspiring leaders. As the other side of the coin is also essential for different insights, I plan to deal with the detrimental aspects of useless leaders in a separate book, perhaps under the lessons learned context considering different use cases for a different audience type. Consequently, I excluded the negative aspects of useless leaders in this book.

Architecting Big Data Solutions Integrated with IoT & Cloud

Create strategic business insights with agility

IoT, Big Data, and Cloud Computing are three distinct technology domains with overlapping use cases. Each technology has its own merits; however, the combination of three creates a synergy and the golden opportunity for businesses to reap the exponential benefits. This combination can create technological magic for innovation when adequately architected, designed, implemented, and operated.

Integrating Big Data with IoT and Cloud architectures provide substantial business benefits. It is like a perfect match. IoT collects real-time data. Big Data optimises data management solutions. Cloud collects, hosts, computes, stores, and disseminates data rapidly.

Based on these compelling business propositions, the primary purpose of this book is to provide practical guidance on creating Big Data solutions integrated with IoT and Cloud architectures. To this end, the book offers an architectural overview, solution practice, governance, and underlying technical approach for creating integrated Big Data, Cloud, and IoT solutions.

The book offers an introduction to solution architecture, three distinct chapters comprising Big Data, Cloud, and the IoT with the final chapter, including conclusive remarks to consider for Big Data solutions. These chapters include essential architectural points, solution practice, methodical rigour, techniques, technologies, and tools.

Creating Big Data solutions are complex and complicated from multiple angles. However, with the awareness and guidance provided in this book, the Big Data solutions architects can be empowered to provide useful and productive solutions with growing confidence.

Digital Intelligence

A framework to digital transformation capabilities

I authored this book because dealing with intelligence, and the digital world is a passion for me and wanted to share my passion with you. In this book, I aim to provide compelling ideas and unique ways to increase, enhance, and deepen your digital intelligence and awareness and apply them to your organisation's digital journey particularly for modernisation and transformation initiatives. I used the architectural thinking approach as the primary framework to convey my message.

Based on my architectural thought leadership on various digital transformation and modernisation engagements, with the accumulated wealth of knowledge and skills, I want to share these learnings in a concise book hoping to add value by contributing to the broader digital community and the progressing initiatives.

Rest assured, this is not a theory or an academic book. It is purely practical and based on lessons learned from real enterprise transformation and modernisation initiatives taken in large corporate environments. I made every effort to make this book concise, uncluttered, and easy-to-read by removing technical jargons for a broader audience who want to enhance digital intelligence and awareness.

Upfront, this book is not about a tool, application, a single product, specific technology, or service, and certainly not to endorse any of these items. However, this book focuses on architectural thinking and methodical approach to improve digital intelligence and awareness. It is not like typical digital transformation books available on the market. In this book, I do not cover and repeat the same content of those books describing digital transformations. My purpose is different.

What distinguishes this book from other books is that I provide an innovative thinking framework and a methodical approach to increase your digital quotient based on experience, aiming not to sell or endorse any products or services even though I mention some prominent technologies which enable digital transformation, for your digital awareness, intelligence, and capabilities.